BHAKTI YOGA

THE YOGA OF DEVOTION!

BESTSELLING AUTHOR

Shreyananda Natha

Cover & Graphic Design

Mattias Långström

Contact: *oneofakindbooks@bhagwan.se*

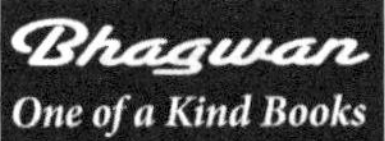

BHAKTI
YOGA

THE YOGA OF DEVOTION!

BESTSELLING AUTHOR

Shreyananda Natha

Copyright © Mattias Långström

ISBN: 9789198735772

✳✳✳

Publisher: **BHAGWAN 2021**

NAMASTÉ

I want to thank the teachers and students I have had over the years and who have made my journey with yoga so interesting. Thank you for all the inspiration you have given me and for making this book possible. The yoga masters who no longer live among us, live on with every new person who immerses themselves in the yoga tradition.

Sri Swami Sivananda, Sri Swami Satyananda, Sri Tirumalai Krishnamacharya, Sri Swami Vishnudevananda, Sri K. Pattabhi Jois, Osho, Swami Nirdosha, Swami Omananda, Swami Janakananda, Ole Schmidt, Turiya, Maryam Abrishami and Sanna Kuittinen.

Everyone who has searched for answers to what they perceived through an activated ajna chakra. In yoga, they have learned the principles behind the universe, the collective consciousness, and the creative power, Kundalini Shakti. The duality behind everything, both what we see and what we do not see. Together we help to pass on the previous secret knowledge, about our gunas, nadis, and chakras, to anyone who wants to be seen.

THE AUTHOR

Shreyananda Natha is the author of over twelve titles on yoga. Among other things, he has written the most comprehensive books on yoga in Swedish – Everything About Yoga and the study book The Yoga Bible. He is also a certified yoga and meditation teacher according to EYTF's international guidelines and has undergone a multi-year yoga teacher training under the leadership of Swami Omananda at Satyananda Ashram. Shreyananda Natha holds the highest initiation in the Tantric Natha Order. He travels frequently to Asia and India to improve himself, and to gain knowledge and inspiration. He has immersed himself in the tantric rituals and is known for his extensive knowledge of yoga, deep relaxation, and meditation

There is no authority that can say what yoga is. When you give yourself fully and completely, and experience yoga without limitations or doubts, when you become one with the true experience in yourself, the real encounter with yoga arises. Only then do you understand what yoga is – for you. You are no longer limited by ornament, shyness and artificial thought patterns that lie as a filter between you and the transformation. Yoga is a cultural-historical wealth that is still passed on from teacher to student and helps man to find his way back to his true nature. It opens us up and attracts awareness. It strengthens our self-esteem, and our entire person's spectrum of possibilities suddenly becomes visible to us. Yoga is not difficult. You do not have to be vegan or able to stand on your head. You just need to practice your yoga regularly and the rest will come by itself.

With all the love from the universe – Aum Shanti/Shreyananda Natha.

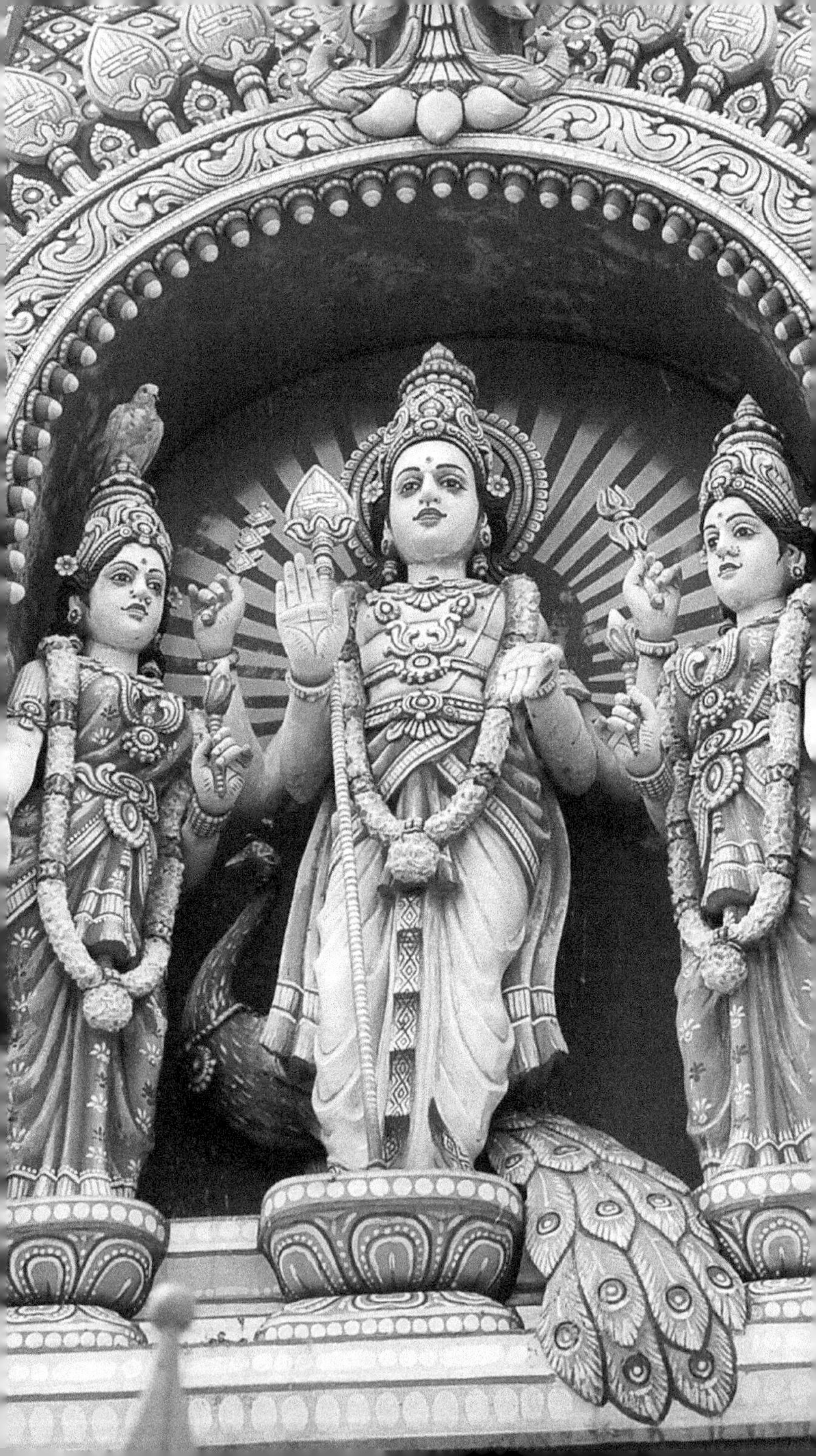

KARMA, BHAKTI & JNANA YOGA

HINDUISM

Hinduism differs from other religions in that it can be described as a collective name for a host of religious denominations that lack a common core. Most Hindus see Hinduism as a set of ritual acts, something practised. But Hinduism is also a tradition that carries a large set of knowledge – it is the religion that has the largest number of sacred texts.

In Hinduism, humans are perceived as thinking, biological and social beings characterized by people's different interests and aptitudes for things. They worship different gods, read different texts, follow different teaching systems and gurus, and visit different temples. This view is the basis for the hierarchical system applied in Hinduism but also the tolerance that exists for each other's differences and diversity.

Diversity expresses the process of change and development that matter, prakriti, undergoes. Purusha, on the other hand, is what all individuals have in common – the unchanging self, the atman, as the samkhya philosophy describes.

Samkhya and yoga both belong to the philosophical system of Hinduism. The purpose of the systems is to guide man towards moksha, or freedom from the cycle of rebirth. Moksha is considered to be the fourth and final goal in a person's life.

The six philosophical systems are arranged in doctrinal pairs as follows:

Nyaya – logic
Vaisheshika – atomic

Samkhya – cosmic principle
Yoga – yoga

Purva-Mimamsa (Vedanta) – ritual
Uttara-Mimamsa (Vedanta) – theological

The belief, within these systems, of a person's own ability to be liberated, differs from the bhakti-oriented theistic Vedan schools, whose adherents believe that a person is dependent on the grace of God to be free from the cycle of rebirth.

Samkhya and yoga are described together in many of the Hindu texts, indicating an early connection to each other.

The Katha, Svetasvatara and Maitri Upanishads describe yogic exercises and samkhya together. In the Katha Upanishad, yoga is used as a means of meditation. Yoga and samkhya are also mentioned in close connection in the Mahabharata. Here, the goal of yoga is described as the realization of the atman (the self) and brahman (matter).

The Bhaghavad Gita, which is part of the Mahabharata, describes yoga in three different ways – jnana, karma and bhakti yoga. Krishna is seen here as the master of yoga.

The Yoga Sutras of Patanjali, an important text in Hinduism, and the most important work of classical yoga, having become and serve as a basic description of it. Here too, samkhya plays a central role. Even yoga traditions that do not share the same view of the ultimate reality have embraced the Yoga Sutras, which describes them logically and coherently. In the Yoga Sutras, yoga is described as the cessation of the activities of the mind, what we today call meditation.

DHARMA

A central concept in Hinduism is dharma, likened to duty, law, rightness and firmness. Many Hindus today call their religion sanatana dharma (the eternal dharma). Dharma is the eternal order, and in the oldest scriptures it refers to the various rituals and duties performed to maintain social and cosmic order.

Dharma is based on the notion that humans maintain the universe through their actions. These actions are covered by various rituals, civil and criminal law, stages of life, pilgrimages, sacrifices, etc. Dharma is used to structure society and the life of the individual. It plays a significant role in the caste systems applied in Hindu society.

Following one's dharma should lead to a better rebirth and be a path to ultimate salvation.

TRADITIONS

The core tradition of Hinduism is brahmanical: the most dominant and widespread tradition in

India. Men in the tradition are authoritarian. The Vedic texts play a central role and are seen as revelations. Within the tradition are the priesthood, a sacred language (Sanskrit) and the perception of a sacred social order. Rituals are performed in temples and ceremonies in the home. Various Hindu deities are worshipped, such as Shiva, Vishnu, Rama, Krishna, Durga, Kali and Ganesha. Pilgrimages, festivals, rules about food and cleanliness are also important.

The other major focus is organizations, where the focus is usually on moksha (salvation). These usually have a founder and some are more ritually oriented (Sri Vishnuism and Sri Vidya), while others function as organizations for ascetics (Vishnuite: Ramanandi and Nada; or Shivaite: Natha and Aghori). They are often bearers of different yoga traditions and men from the Brahmin class are often seen as leaders of these groups.

The guru movements also belong to this tradition; these often have to compete for followers. Many have also succeeded in communicating their teachings internationally such as Maharishi Mahesh Yogi (Transcendental Meditation) and A.C. Bhaktivedanta Swami Prabhupada (International Society for Krishna Consciousness).

A third focus is the village and tribe-based traditions of India. Priests in this tradition are not from the Brahmin class and gods who have a local connection are worshipped. The Brahmin core tradition sees these practices as unclean, which has led to a tense relationship.

VISHNUISM, SHIVAISM AND SHAKTISM

Sacrifice rituals were a central part of the brahmanic tradition, but became less important as the ascetic ideology emerged. Knowledge and renunciation became more important than being freed from the cycle of rebirth. Many of the gods who were important in the Vedic sacrificial tradition fell away, while Shiva and Vishnu remain important. Groups sprang up where one of these gods was worshipped, laying the foundation for Hinduism as a religion. The ritual worship of gods (puja) that then arose competed with the sacrificial culture (yajna).

Seventy per cent of Hindus worship Vishnu or one of his avatars, such as Rama or Krishna. Vishnu's task is to sustain the world. In the

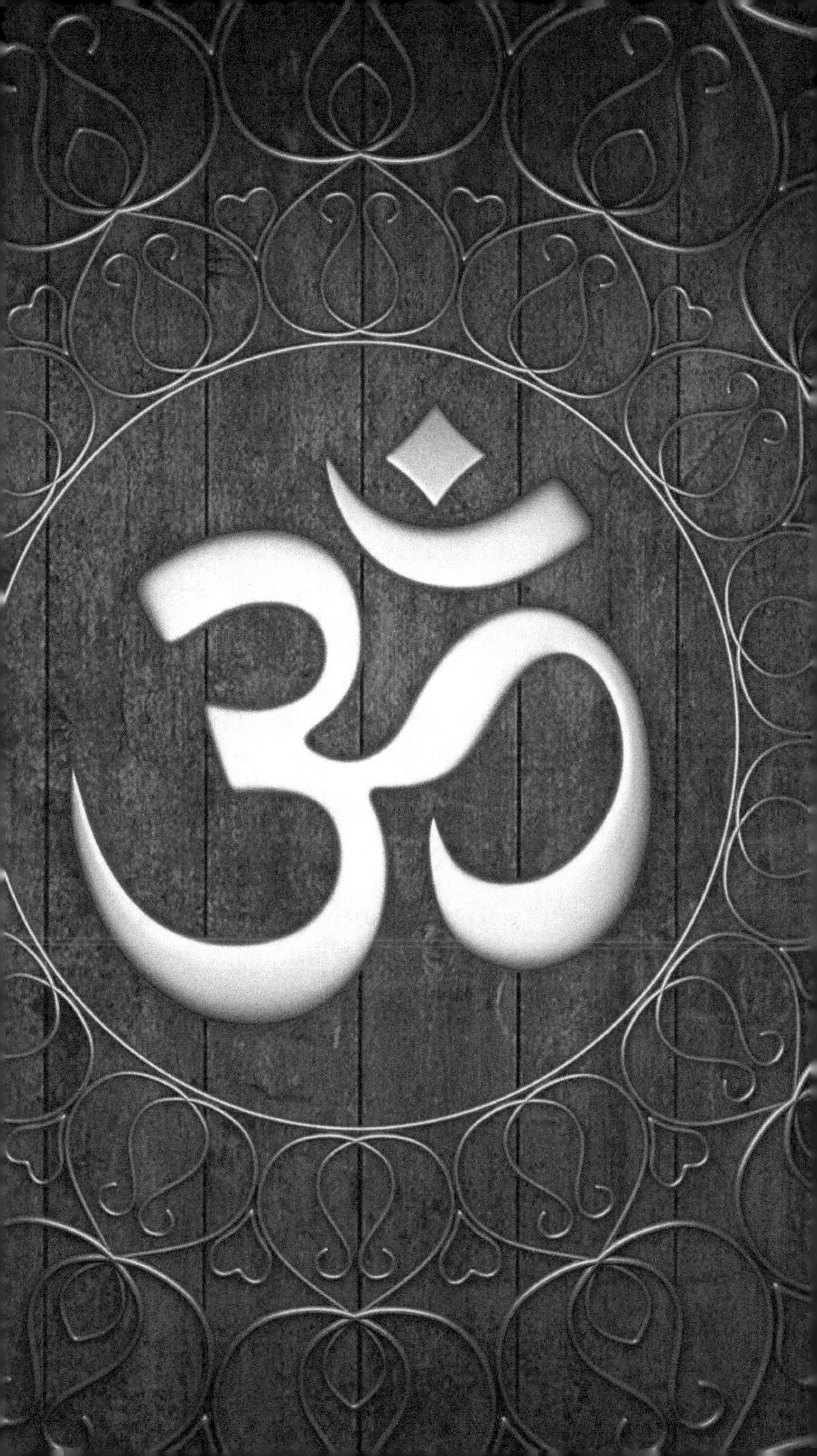

form of Krishna, he evokes feelings of love and care. In the form of Rama, he symbolizes the world order, dharma and the dutiful man. Worship and devotion to a personal god is what characterizes Vishnuism, but there are also organizations for ascetics and some groups have taken up some of tantrism and instead worship a goddess such as Lakshmi.

Twenty-eight per cent of Hindus worship Shiva and his family members, his wife Parvati and their sons Ganesha and Skanda. Shiva is the great yogi and a friendly god, but also has sides where he appears dangerous, destructive and terrible. Shivaism is common in the Himalayan region and is largely yogic. Some Hindu ascetics also worship him.

The 13th to 16th centuries were a great time for Shivaite ascetics and Natha yogis in northern India. They practised hatha yoga and various tantric rituals. Gorakhnatha is the most famous Natha yogi. He was a student of Matsyendranatha, who himself was a disciple of Siva. Through hatha yoga, one could stop the decay of the body and activate kundalini Shakti, to create an immortal body that would lead to

the Shiva state. According to Natha yogis, only
hatha yoga could lead to this condition; other
religious paths were considered unnecessary.

About two per cent of Hindus follow Shaktism
and worship the goddess Shakti, the female
power of the supreme divine principle. She
is seen as the ultimate reality (brahman), the
creative power (Shakti), the matter in creation
(prakriti), the one who hides (maya) and the
saviour. Shaktism has evolved from Shivaism.
Many female figures were found during the
excavations in the Indus Valley, although it is
unclear what they represented. It was not until
the seventh century AD, that Shaktism was
mentioned in the written traditions.

Female ideology also plays a central role in tantrism, whose concept is based on the belief that
our external environment and our bodies consist
of both female and male aspects, and that
salvation comes through uniting this polarity.
To achieve tantric salvation (sadhana), mantras, mudras, nyasa and puja are used. Tantrism
combines jnana and karma yoga. Knowledge
is what ultimately saves a person and action is
what gives them experience of the ultimate rea-

lity. Kundalini yoga was developed as a separate branch of yoga within tantrism and is based on the goddess ideology of tantrism and Shaktism. The path of tantrism is the most effective for the world we live in today, the Kali era. Old techniques are more difficult to apply.

HINDUISM AND YOGA

In the 1920s, archaeological excavations were made along the Indus River and uncovered the remains of the two large cities, Mohenjo Daro and Harappa. Both yoga and Hinduism most likely originate from this era, when the Indus and Saraswati civilizations existed.

The excavations also uncovered fall-stones, which are an important symbol of the god Shiva, and signets, one of which depicted a person with animal horns sitting in a meditation position surrounded by four animals. Shiva is often called the master of animals, which may indicate that he was already being worshipped when the Indus culture flourished between 5,000 and 3,000 BC. Shiva is called the great yogi, which indicates that yoga's origins were from this time.

Modern technology has helped to establish that the river Saraswati dried up sometime during the 30th century BC. In the Rigveda, the river Saraswati is praised, suggesting this sacred text must have come into being earlier. Yoga is mentioned in the Rigveda, indicating that it too probably originated before the 30th century BC.

Yoga plays a central role in Hinduism and is used as a method of physical and mental discipline as well as to achieve spiritual salvation. It is the part of Hinduism that most people have experienced – both Hindus and non-Hindus. The original goal of yoga in the Hindu tradition is to reach salvation or enlightenment with the help of the body, using various physical and mental techniques. In the West, yoga has mostly been used to strengthen the body and find peace. Like Hinduism, yoga is also pluralistic, which means that there are many different types of physical and mental exercises depending on which tradition you choose.

Traditions can define the concept of yoga in different ways. The most common translation among Hindus is "union", which refers to a union between body and soul. In the Patanjali

Yoga Sutras, one of the most important texts in yoga, it is defined as yoga chitta vritti nirodhah, or cessation of the activities of the mind.

Within the yoga traditions, the term yoga has five main meanings:

1.A disciplined method of achieving a goal.

2.A technique for controlling the body.

3. A name for one of the six philosophical systems of Hinduism.

4. In combination with other words such as hatha, mantra and laya, yoga refers to traditions that have focused on specific yoga techniques.

5. Objectives for the practice of yoga.

Central to any tradition is breathing and breath control. Holding the breath is considered in the brahmanic tradition as a ritual act. Atharvaveda tells of breathing and its connection to the body's energies. The Chandogya Upanishad describes five different types of breathing, the inner sound and the nadis.

YOGA AND BUDDHISM

Buddhism has its roots in Indian yoga and was from its beginning a form of yoga. The Buddha himself was taught by yoga teachers and his experiences became the basis of the Buddhist meditation doctrine. Buddhist yoga and Hindu yoga are thus closely related and may have influenced each other for many hundreds of years. Concepts such as nirodha/nirvana (cessation) and dukha (suffering) are common to both traditions. The Buddhist eight-fold path and Indian eight-fold yoga have many similarities. The big difference is that in Indian yoga the body and breathing have a much greater significance. The most important goal in both traditions is to put an end to avidya, false knowledge.

The Scriptures of Veda
Veda means knowledge and the scriptures are divided into four parts (samitha):

1. The Rigveda (roughly the 30th century BC) is the oldest part of the Vedic scriptures, where yoga and the Saraswati river are mentioned. These vedas are hymns that are recited and serve as regulations for various rituals. In order to perform the rituals successfully, various yoga

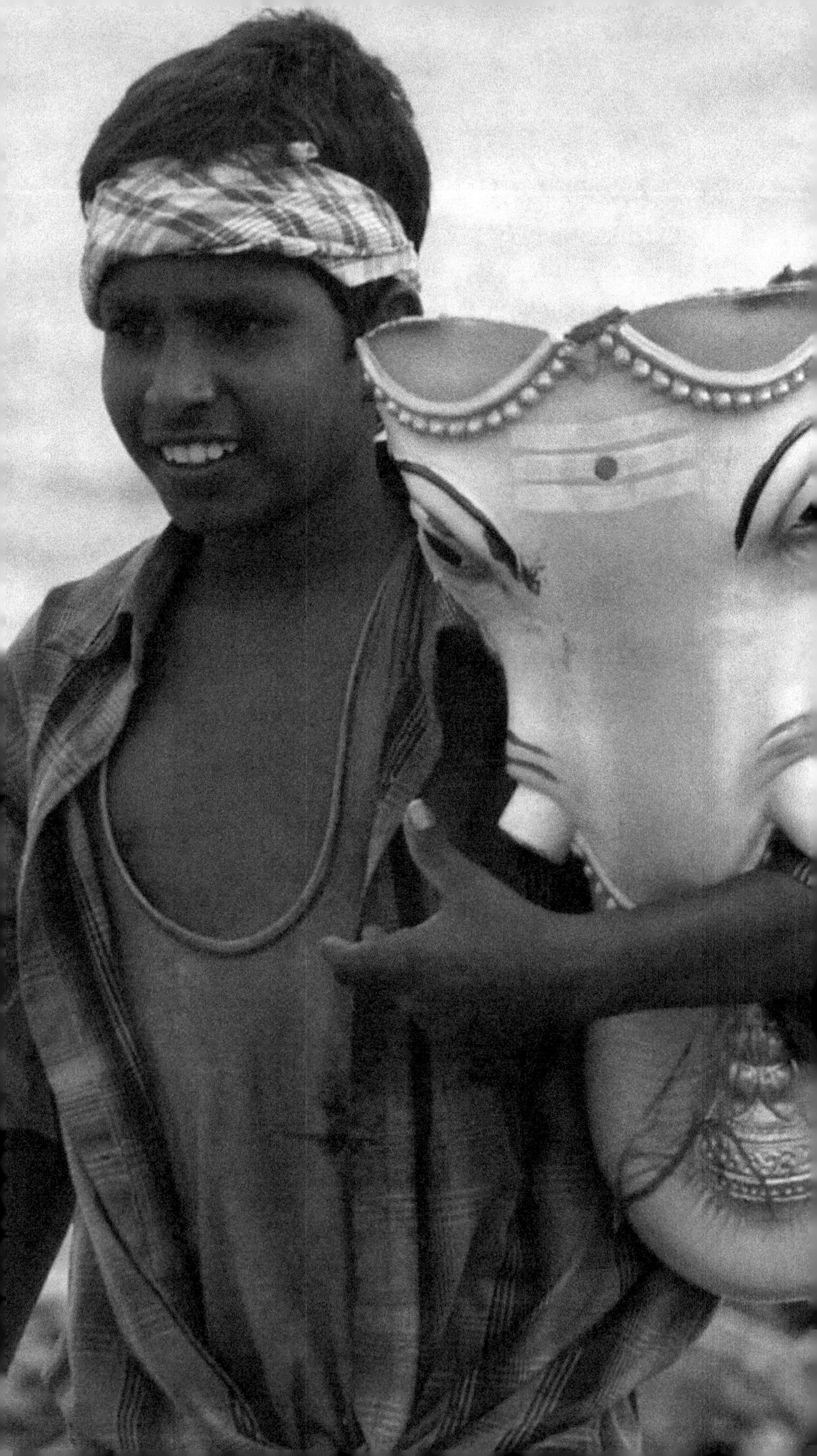

techniques were developed to strengthen the ability to concentrate.

2. The Samaveda are vedas with sung hymns.

3. The Yajurveda are vedas with ritual texts.

4. The Atharvaveda are vedas with magic formulas.

According to the Vedic worldview, our world is a reflection of the cosmic world. By maintaining the cosmic order in our world, one can create a harmonious existence. To get an inner picture of the cosmic order, followers use various yoga techniques such as regulated breathing, mantra singing and concentration exercises.

These samithas are the first part of the wood. Three more texts are included:

1. Brahmana: comments on the vedas that explain the rituals of each samitha.

2. Aranyaka: "Forest books".

3. The Upanishads: The last part of the vedas

and often seen as the most important. This esoteric text describes the worldview found in Vedanta and is the most famous philosophical system in India.

The Upanishads are based on four basic concepts:

1. That the brahman (world soul) is identical to the atman (the human soul), which means that the creative energy of the universe is identical to our inner self.

2. The realization that the unity of everything leads to spiritual enlightenment – moksha. This insight frees us from the cycle of rebirth.

3. The law of karma, which means that our thoughts and actions affect our future.

4. If you do not reach insight, you are born according to your karma.

In the Katha, Svetasvarata and Maitri Upanishads you can find descriptions of yoga exercises as well as samkhya concepts and performances, which indicates that yoga has been associated with samkhya from an early age.

"It is the highest state: When the five sense organs and the mind have calmed down and the intellect is immobile. This control of the senses they call yoga. Then he is free from disturbances, for yoga is both origin and cessation."

(Katha-Upanishad 6.10-11)

"By holding the body with its top three parts right and get the feelings and senses to go in the heart, the sage crosses all dangerous rivers with Brahman as boat.

While controlling breathing and all movements, he should breathe through his nose, with controlled breathing sounds the wise control his mind as he steer a chariot drawn by wild horses.

In an even and clean place, free from pebbles, fire and sand, near running water, in one place the mind finds attractive and to which the eye does not react as ugly, in a hidden place sheltered from the wind, he should practice yoga."

(Svetasvatara-Upanishad 2.8-2.10)

THE MAHABHARATA

Yoga is also mentioned in the Mahabharata, which belongs to the category of itihasa (history) and which is one of two great epic works in Hinduism, especially in Books 12 and 13 where, yoga is described in close connection with samkhya:

> "WHAT YOGIS SEE IS THE SAME AS THE FOLLOWERS OF SAMKHYA PERCEIVE. HE IS A SAGE WHO SEES SAMKHYA AND YOGA AS THE SAME."
>
> (MAHABHARATA 12.293.30)

The Bhagavad Gita is a mythological work of poetry and the most important scripture in bhakti yoga. This great epic belongs to the Mahabharata and was added about 700 AD. It is seen as a summary of the Upanishads. Here, Krishna is described as the master of yoga, and yoga is seen as a disciplined method of achieving a goal. Three yoga paths are described – jnana, karma and bhakti, of which bhakti is seen as the highest.

"It is better to follow one's own dharma badly than another's flawlessly."

(Baghavad Gita 3.35)

"While sitting there, he should practice yoga to clear the mind, keep the mind attached to an object and restrain the mind and emotions. activity."

(Baghavad Gita 6.12)

DIFFERENT YOGA PATHS

As said, yoga is a broad tradition with many branches and techniques. Down the ages, masters have developed various techniques for spiritual enlightenment. There are no direct boundaries between the yoga paths, but everyone goes in some way into each. Within a yoga tradition, one can use many different techniques.

KARMA YOGA – THE WAY OF ACTION

Karma yoga is the way of action and is mainly suitable for people who are outgoing in nature. It means working, performing social activities and helping other people with no thought of getting anything in return. Karma yoga is a continuation of the Vedic sacrificial doctrine where sacrifices were made to the gods. In the Bhagavad Gita, sacrificial acts mean one is loyal to the doctrine of warning, that they follow their dharma and the class they belong to.

Today, karma yoga is more about selfless, moral action. The job itself is not the most important, but rather one's attitude during its execution. One's attitude determines whether the action or job is perceived as liberating or binding, painful and hard. Whatever you choose to do, make

sure you always do your best. If you can do the
job better, you make sure to do it. One should
not let negative thoughts hold one back, such as
fear of criticism. You should also not feel bound
by or dependent on your job, but be prepared
to leave it if necessary. Mahatma Gandhi and
Mother Teresa are two famous karma yogis.

BHAKTI YOGA – THE WAY OF DEDICATION

This path is suitable for people who are emotio-
nal with nature. One surrenders oneself to God
through prayers, worship and rituals, driven
by the power of love and experiencing God as
love itself. Being devoted and loving towards a
personal god is considered to lead to salvation.
Chanting and singing God's name is a central
part of bhakti yoga.

RAJA YOGA – THE WAY OF MEDITATION

Often called the royal way, raja yoga involves
the control of thoughts. One trains the mind
through meditation and transforms mental and
physical energy into spiritual energy. Raja yoga
is also called ashtanga yoga, which refers to
"eight-step yoga", which should systematically
lead to control of the mind. When the body and
energy are under control and in harmony, meditation takes place by itself.

Ashtanga yoga's eight steps – the Yoga Sutras of
Patanjali:

1. Yamas – five basic ideas about moral discipline, "do not do":

Ahimsa – do not use violence.
Sathyam – be true.
Brahmacharya – moderation, control over desi-
re, chastity.
Asteya – do not steal.
Aparighara – do not be greedy.

2. Niyamas – five basic ideas about ethical action, "should do":

Saucha – external and internal cleanliness, such
as thoughts, speech, hygiene.
Santosha – contentment.
Tapas – restraint, self–discipline.
Swadhyaya – studies.
Ishvara pranidhana – the worship of God.

3. Asana – body position.
The lotus position. To be able to sit completely
immobile so as not to be distracted by the physical body during meditation.

4. Pranayamas – controlled breathing.
Controlled breathing to control the pran in the
body, which calms the mind.

5. Pratyahara – directs the sense organs inward.
Calms the mind when you are not disturbed by
the environment and external stimuli.

6. Dharana – concentration.
Concentration is achieved by focusing on an
object.

7. Dhyana – meditation.
After a long period of concentration, meditation
is achieved.

8. Samadhi – ecstasy.
Prolonged meditation leads to ecstasy. The yogi
becomes at one with the object of meditation
when the movements of the mind cease.

JNANA YOGA – THE WAY OF KNOWLEDGE
This is perhaps the most difficult path because it
requires a strong will and a sharp intellect. It is
mainly suitable for people who are theoretically
inclined. A jnana yogi comes to an understan-
ding of the transient and the eternal in life by

studying Vedanta, which belong to the Upanishads, the last part of the Vedic scriptures. It is
difficult to reach spiritual insight through theo-
retical knowledge; therefore, it is important
to practise other yoga paths as a preparation.
Ramana Maharishi is a well-known jnana yogi.

THE MANTRA

The mantra consists of words and syllables that
carry a special vibration and affect the mind
and body in a positive and strengthening way.
According to tradition, mantras have been used
to reach a deeper plane of consciousness.

With mantra meditation you calm your thoughts
and mind. By repeating the same mantra over
and over again, you do not give the mind any
new stimulus, instead allowing the subconscious mind to wake up. Old thoughts and memories
have an opportunity to come to the surface and
the subconscious mind can be purified from
them. One looks more clearly at life and is no
longer governed by old thought patterns. In the
same way that asanas are meant to strengthen
and purify the body, the mantra is meant to
calm and "clean up" the mind.

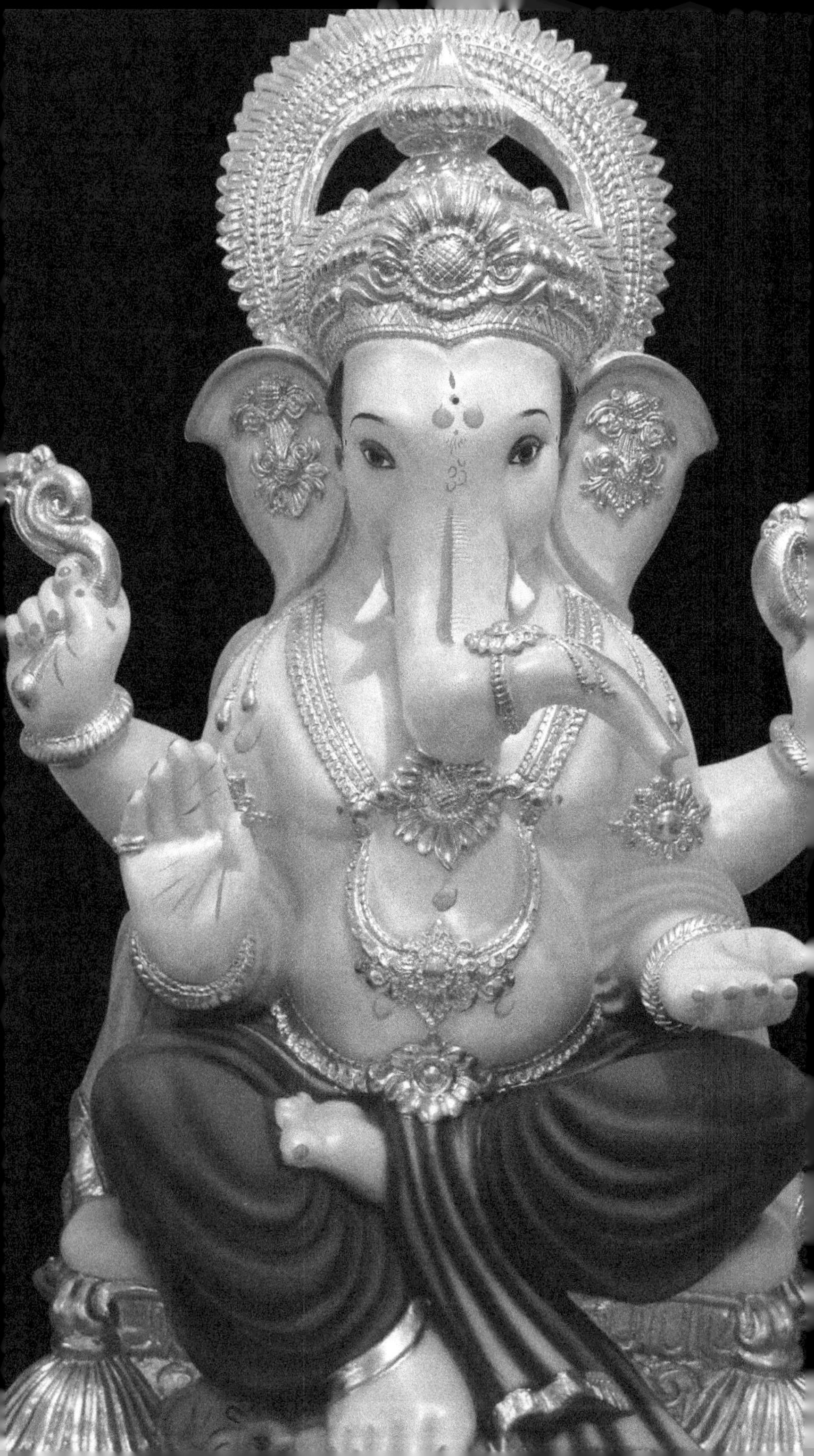

In yoga, it is believed that everything in the universe consists of energy that vibrates differently. Mantras consist of a high vibration that should have a beneficial and positive effect on our body. When we recite or sing a mantra, we begin to vibrate at the same rate. In our palate we have eighty-four meridian points that affect the pituitary gland, the pineal gland and the chemical balance of the brain. When we pronounce certain mantras, the tongue hits these meridian points, which can increase mental clarity and awareness.

Most often one recites a mantra one hundred and eight times. Our physical and subtle body has seventy-two thousand energy channels called nadis. One hundred and eight of these meet at hrit padma, the area around the anahata chakra. By repeating a mantra one hundred and eight times, the whole physical and subtle body is permeated by its energy.

THE GAYATRI MANTRA

The gayatri mantra is said to be the oldest mantra, with its origins in the Rigveda Vedic scripture. It is sometimes called savitri, because in the mantra one prays to Deva Savitr, the sun god who was worshipped during the Vedic period (the sun before sunrise is called savitri and after sunrise surya). The gayatri mantra is also found in other Hindu texts such as the Bhagavad Gita, and is of great importance in the Hindu traditions. It is taught to children when they turn eight years old.

The gayatri mantra is said to heal physically, mentally and emotionally. It expands consciousness, promotes spiritual development and develops one's intellectual potential, knowledge and wisdom. It seems sattvic.

THE GAYATRI MANTRA
Om bhur bhuvaha svaha
Tat savitur varenyam
Bhargo devasya dhimahi
Dhiyo yonah prachodayat

"Praise to the source of all things.
It is due to you that we attain true
happiness on the planes of earth,
astral, casual. It is due to your
transcendent nature that you are
worthy of being worshiped and
adored. Ignite us with your all
pervading light"

THE MAHAMRITYUNJAYA MANTRA

This mantra also has its roots in the Rigveda Vedic literature, and is also called the tryambakam mantra. It is dedicated to "the three-eyed": an epithet of Rudra, who later came to be characterized as Shiva.

The mahamrityunjaya mantra provides peace and protection. It is said to heal physically, mentally and emotionally. It counteracts rajas.

THE MAHAMRITYUNJAYA MANTRA

Om triambakam yajamahe
Sugandhim pushti vardanam
Urvarukamiva bandhanan
Mrityor muksheeya mamritat

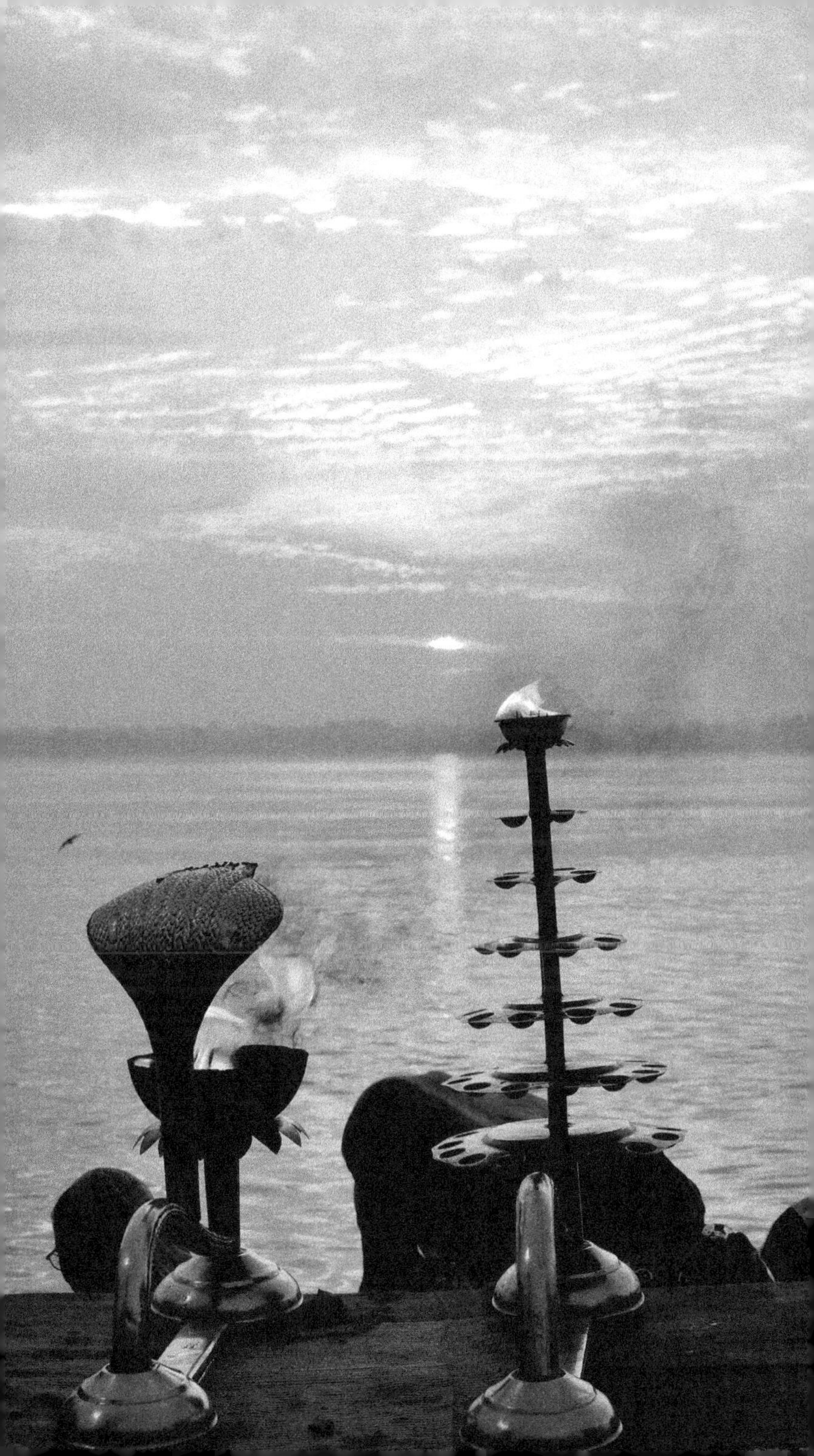

"Shelter me, the three-eyed Lord Shiva. Bless me with health and immortality and sever me from the clutches of death, even as a cucumber is cut from its creeper"

THE INFLUENCE OF TANTRISM ON YOGA

During the post-classical period, it was primarily tantrism that came to influence the yoga tradition.

According to tantrism, the divine power (kundalini Shakti) in the human body is inactive. This brings the physical body into focus for the ritual exercises, a new phenomenon in the spiritual history of India.

THE BHAGAVAD GITA

The Bhagavad Gita (the "Song of God") is the god Krishna's song. It is a mythological work in Sanskrit, and an independent story in the great epic, the Mahabharata. In the Bhagavad Gita, a dialogue takes place between Krishna and Prince Arjuna, just before the great battle of Kurukshetra. Arjuna faces a difficult dilemma: his duty as a warrior is to follow his dharma and begin the battle, but at the same time he sees it as a terrible sin to kill the many great men, relatives and gurus who are in the opponents' army. To accompany the prince through this difficult decision, Krishna teaches him various forms of yoga. The story takes place about five thousand years ago.

The Bhagavad Gita can be seen as a summary of the Upanishads. Each chapter ends with the Bhagavad Gita being called Upanishad.

Krishna says in Bhagavad Gita 3.3 that there have been two paths since ancient times:

Karma yoga – the way of action, that is to do one's duty without worrying about the outcome.

Jnana yoga – the way of knowledge, that is knowledge of the self (atman).

Other ways are variants of these.

Krishna shows his vishvarupa, his universal form, for Arjuna on the battlefield at Kurukshetra.

The Bhagavad Gita consists of eighteen chapters:

1. Arjuna lets Krishna pull his chariot to a place in the middle of the two armies. When Arjuna sees his relatives on the opposite side of Kurus, he loses his motivation and decides not to fight.

2. Krishna explains to Arjuna that his concern about fighting against his relatives and gurus is unjustified, because only the body can be killed, while the eternal self is immortal. Krishna reminds Arjuna that as a warrior he has a duty to follow, his dharma, and wage war.

3. Arjuna asks why he has to fight if knowledge is more important than action. Krishna emphasizes that the right way to act is to carry out one's duties for good, but without clinging to the results.

4. Krishna says that he has lived through many births and always taught yoga to protect the righteous and to annihilate the unrighteous. He emphasizes the importance of trusting a guru.

5. Arjuna asks Krishna if it is better to refrain from action or to perform actions. Krishna replies that both ways can be good, but that action, karma yoga, is the highest.

6. Krishna describes the correct position of meditation and the process of achieving samadhi.

7. Krishna teaches the way of knowledge, jnana yoga.

8. Krishna defines the terms brahman, adhyatma, karma, atman, adhibhuta and adhidaiva, and explains how to remember him at the moment of death and attain a higher state.

9. Krishna describes panentheism, "all beings are in me", as a way of remembering him in all circumstances.

10. Krishna declares that he is the ultimate source of all material and spiritual worlds. Arjuna recognizes Krishna as the supreme being, and quotes famous scholars who have done the same.

11. At Arjuna's request, Krishna demonstrates a theophany, its "universal form", Visvarupa: a terrifying creature that is turned in all directions at the same time, which spreads the radiation from a thousand suns around it, and which contains all other beings and all matter that exists.

12. Krishna describes the process of devotion, bhakti yoga.

13. Krishna describes matter (prakriti) and consciousness (purusha).

14. Krishna talks about the three states, gunas, which together constitute all beings.

15. Krishna describes a symbolic tree, which represents the material existence, its roots in heaven and its foliage on earth. He explains that this tree should be felled with the "axe of indifference" so that one can move on to a higher state.

16. Krishna describes the human traits of divine and demonic beings. He advises that the higher state can be achieved by renouncing lust, anger and greed and by distinguishing right actions from wrong deeds through buddhi and advice from scriptures and thereby acting right.

17. Krishna talks about the three variants of faith, of knowledge, of actions, and even of eating habits, which are linked to the three gunas.

18. In conclusion, Krishna asks Arjuna to abandon all dharma and solely submit to him. He describes this as the ultimate and final perfection of life.

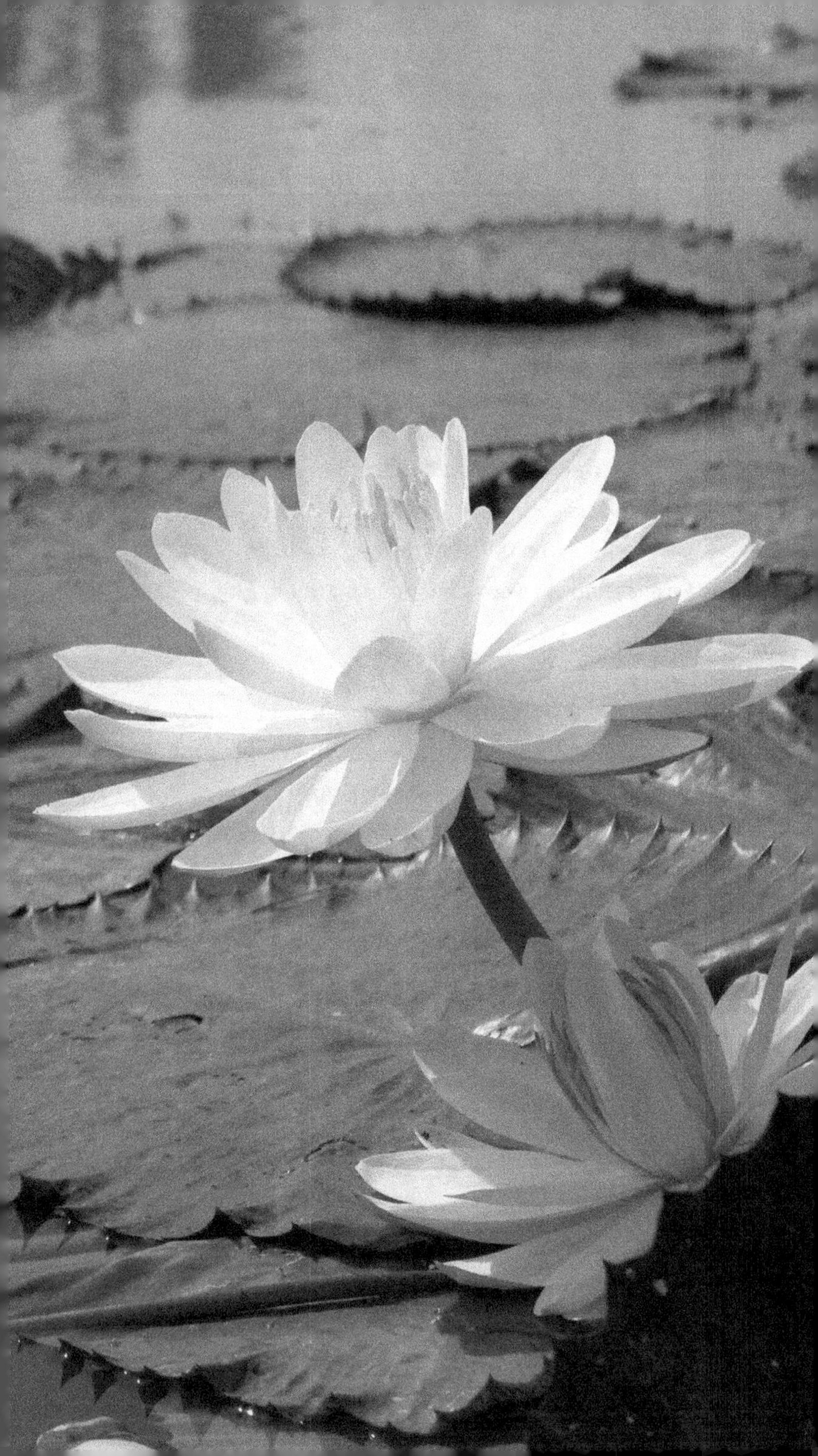

www.ingramcontent.com/pod-product-compliance
Lightning Source LLC
La Vergne TN
LVHW041245200726
843507LV00013B/2822